I0468528

Raw Food Diet for Beginners

Seven Easy Steps for Nutrition, Health and Vitality

Introduction

I want to thank you and congratulate you for downloading the book, *Raw Food Diet for Beginners: Seven Easy Tips for Nutrition, Health and Vitality.*

This book contains proven steps and strategies on how to transition from a standard diet to a raw food alternative. A raw food diet means only eating foods that haven't been cooked- just like it sounds like! However, following a raw food diet also strongly recommends not eating anything processed or pasteurized, as well as eating only organic foods. For this book, we'll be assuming that all of the above are true when we talk about raw foods.

So what is the benefit of a raw food diet anyway? We're glad you asked! When food is cooked, a lot of the natural enzymes found within the food are lost. These enzymes normally aid in digestion, making cooked food, therefore, harder for us to digest. With a raw food diet, digestion has never been easier. Our body can focus less energy on digestion and more energy on absorbing the vitamins, minerals, and other nutrients of the food. The end result is that your very cells are cleaner and function better, leading to a boost in nutrition, health, and vitality!

Keep in mind that raw food technically means you'll be eating a vegetarian diet. Since you can't eat anything cooked or processed, most every type of meat becomes unavailable for consumption. Don't let that scare you away! With proper transitioning tactics and some good recipes, you won't even miss the foods you have to give up. If nutrition, health, and vitality are your priorities, the raw food option is really your best choice- even devout carnivores should give it a shot!

Thanks again for downloading this book, I hope you enjoy it!

not allowed unless with written permission from the publisher. All rights reserved.

permission or backing by the trademark owner. All trademarks and brands within this book are for clarifying purposes only and are the owned by the owners themselves, not affiliated with this document.

Table of Contents

Chapter 1: Get Educated 8

Chapter 2: Be Goal Oriented 12

Chapter 3: Start Slow 17

Chapter 4: Outfit Your Kitchen 21

Chapter 5: Check Out Local Food Options 26

Chapter 6: Moderate and Track Your Nutrition 31

Chapter 7: Keep Up the Exercise 36

Chapter 1- Educate Yourself!

You might be thinking to yourself, 'well that's why I'm here!' And you're absolutely right! However, this book is focused on allowing people with a standard diet to transition into a raw food diet naturally and healthily. While we will be doing our very best to educate you along every step of the way, you still might find yourself in need of some extra learning. There are a couple reasons why you might need to learn more about raw food diets. If you are unsure whether raw foods are for you or if you have a specific dietary concern, it would be in your best interest to look for a little extra information on the side. Don't go now, though! In the meantime, we'll give your education a jump-start.

First, let's start with how the raw food movement originated. The history of the raw food movement is a storied one, with the earliest noted practitioner dating back to 1830. A Presbyterian Minister thought raw foods to be the cure for many ailments and began to preach for the consumption of raw foods. While some of his tenants may have been misguided (he believed raw foods curbed one's lust, for example), this minister is one of the earliest documented proponents of the diet and helped to cement the idea in the masses of age past. More recently, author Weston A. Price observed dental and jaw degeneration within one generation of people who stopped eating nutrient rich, raw foods. In his travels, he noted that the tribes with the healthiest dental structures all had a large percentage of raw food in their diet. His 1939 work, *Nutrition and Physical Degradation,* heralded a wave of raw food activists in the 20th century. Finally, it was one Leslie Kenton and her book *Raw Energy- Eat Your Way to Radiant Health* that finally pushed raw foods to the forefront of our minds. In this book, Kenton recommended sprouts, seeds, and vegetable juices- all veritable stapes of the raw food kitchen.

Now that you know a bit more about the origin of raw food, let's take a look at some people that may not take to raw foods quite as well. If you're planning on also going vegan with your raw food diet, then some people may be concerned with nutritional deficiencies. Children are the most susceptible to possible deficiencies. Raw food diets may not contain enough vitamin b12 or vitamin D to support a healthy child's diet. Before you put your children on a raw food diet, consult your doctor or a dietician about how the best way to plan and transition from a standard diet. Another subset of people that might have difficulty with raw food diets include people suffering from anorexia or diabetes, as well as other individuals with very specific dietary needs. As with children, consult with a doctor or dietician if you feel you might be at risk. Most grown adults with healthy lifestyles will suffer no problems whatsoever from switching to a raw food diet- in fact, their nutrition, health, and vitality will markedly improve!

You may be asking, 'where do I go from here?' The first steps are to make sure you're fully aware of what a raw food diet entails and that your lifestyle will be able to encompass that effectively. Once you've figured that out, there's a lot of research that can raise the effectiveness of your diet. Looking up delicious recipes is a great start! You might also consider looking into seminars or meet-ups that discuss the raw food movement in your local area. As we will discuss later in the book, looking for local food options such as a farmers market is also a must. As you continue reading through this book, it would be a good idea to keep a notebook nearby in order to write down things you might want to look into in the future. Remember, a raw food diet is paramount to your nutrition, health, and vitality, so you want to be as educated as possible about what you're eating as you press forth into uncharted waters!

Chapter 2- Be Goal Oriented

Every type of raw food diet will help you achieve nutrition, health, and vitality- that much is a fact! However, raw food diets can also help you in a number of other realms. In addition to striving for better health, you can also tailor your raw food diet to assist with weight loss or detoxification of the body. By modifying the types of foods you focus on as well as food preparation, you can achieve any or all of these positive benefits! In this chapter, we will look at these three focuses and provide a number of tips and steps that can help anyone achieve these goals.

First, let's talk about raw food for better health. Many people that are reading this book are simply interested in leading a healthier lifestyle. Well, you're on your way- this book is an excellent first step! As we've already outlined above, raw food diets allow your body to absorb more nutrients from every bite of food, maximizing the healthy aspects of your food and minimizing the stress on your digestive system. Eating any kind of raw food diet is going to be good for your health, but what if you want to go that extra mile and really focus on vibrant, clean vitality? For the best pro-health results, the absolute most important step is to eat organic foods. While this is important for all raw food diets, organic foods provide the untampered nutrients and lack of pesticides and preservatives that your body craves. Vegan diets are also a great option to reach the absolute pinnacle of health. Lastly, look into the recently touted super foods such as kale, chia seeds, and kefir.

Secondly, we'll look into the best way to use raw food as a weight-loss mechanism. Raw foods are naturally less fattening than many processed and cooked foods, and many people will find that losing weight on a raw food diet is easier than they could have imagined! Simply by virtue of switching to the diet, you're already cutting out a huge amount of fats, sugars, and salty foods that can easily plump you up. In this way, many people don't find that they need to put any extra effort into losing weight while eating a raw food diet. Your body naturally digests and uses every little bit of raw food much better than processed foods with a ton of excess, indigestible waste. Because of this, your body operates much more cleanly and effectively, with less of a need to store fats. However, if you're really adamant about putting away those pounds, focus on drinking lots of water and eating alkaline-rich foods.

Lastly, we'll take a look at eating raw foods in order to detoxify your body. Detoxing is a process that removes toxins and other residual, harmful materials that can become stored in your fat and cells. Just like the weight loss method, the

detox method of raw food diets will rely heavily on alkaline foods and super foods. You'll want to drink plenty of green vegetable juices and eat as many superfoods as you can such as blueberries, acai berries, and goji berries. Wheatgrass powder and foods that are high in amino acids are also great for this method. Detoxification will help you get rid of all the toxins that have built up in your body from a standard diet, and will make your raw food diet much more effective afterward. With detoxing, lots of water and exercise arc an absolute must as well!

To conclude, raw food diets are very versatile. If you're looking for a specific dietary benefit, it's likely that a raw food diet can provide it. Raw foods are especially good for weight loss and detoxifying your body. Many people lose weight simply by virtue of switching to the diet, while the mineral-rich, natural foods are also incredibly helpful for removing harmful substances built up in the cells and fat stores. Of course, raw food is perfect for an all-around health-conscious diet as well. Whatever you're looking for out of a diet, chances are that raw food is the way to go!

Chapter 3- Start Slow

Many people can find transitioning to a raw food diet somewhat difficult. In this day and age, many people tend to eat out a lot, consuming fast foods and pre-prepared foods almost daily. For many of us, the idea of cutting out cooked and processed foods seems impossible. Don't worry, feeling like this is normal! Rather than cutting out everything all at once, many people find that it's much easier to slowly transition from a standard diet to a raw food diet. This way, you can figure out what works for you. Some people prefer a mix of raw foods and the standard diet. While a pure raw food diet is your absolute best bet for nutrition, health, and vitality, it is important to find what works for you before committing to a new diet.

To start off, take a couple weeks slowly integrating raw foods into your diet. A good way to start is to replace your snacks with raw food alternatives. Instead of snacking on potato chips or candy, try snacking on nut mixes and dried fruit. Once you've grown comfortable with those changes,

you can then start switching around meal choices. Cut out the cooked meat in your meals for lentils, beans, and nuts. This is the time during your transition in which looking up some delicious recipes will be beneficial. When transitioning, it becomes very important that you find something that your taste buds love as much as your body does. A lot of people have the misconception that vegan, vegetarian, and indeed raw food diets give up taste for

health. That simply isn't true! The internet provides a

wealth of wonderful resources for making your food just

as delicious as you'd like it to be. This is really a more

important aspect than most people think, so take some

time and do the research. Don't be afraid to try new

things. Once you've reconciled your new diet with your

palate, you'll be well on your way to a full raw food diet

with a stomach as happy as your body!

This period is where you will really be deciding which level of raw foods works best for you. While everybody should strive for a 100% raw, vegan diet, the fact of the matter is that this dietary style simply doesn't work for everybody. If a completely raw food diet isn't for you, don't feel bad! Even having a 30% raw diet is incredibly beneficial to your health. Most people that practice this diet find themselves around the 75%-80% mark, which is completely acceptable. When transitioning, there are a couple important things you want to keep in mind. Weigh out the pros and cons as you see them. As you're transitioning, trust your taste buds. After trying a number of different options, if most of what you taste is unsatisfying or doesn't taste good, then raw food may simply not be the best option for you. On the plus side, appreciate the simplicity of the diet. Because the food is uncooked, the preparation of raw food meals is usually a lot quicker and easier than cooked meals.

In conclusion, go slow and be mindful. If you take your time transitioning from a standard to a raw food diet and make sure you pay attention to how your body, taste palate, and fullness react, you're guaranteed to find what balance of raw and cooked foods works best for you. There is a fine line to walk here between experimentation and trusting your gut. A lot of people have never had any experience eating exclusively raw foods, so it is entirely possible that they may suffer a taste backlash at first. This is why we recommend transitioning snacks first. These small, mini-meals give you a chance to sample a wide variety of different foods. You'll get a chance to determine what tastes you like and don't like, without giving up your major meals just yet. It is during this step that many people are able to feel out exactly how much of a change they would like to make. If you take your time and aren't afraid to try new things, we guarantee you'll be able to make raw foods work for you!

Chapter 4- Outfit Your Kitchen

One of the most important aspects of transitioning to a raw food diet is making sure that your kitchen is up to snuff. While the actual preparation of many raw foods is delightfully simple compared to cooked food alternatives, there is a good deal of specialized equipment that will make your raw food experience that much better. This chapter will focus on how to rework your kitchen so that you have the best raw food preparation area available!

To outfit your kitchen, start by cleaning, organizing, and minimizing. This is a great time to give your kitchen a deep clean. Use whatever methods are normally preferable to you, but try using biodegradable and organic cleaning solutions. It's a great way to symbolically set your kitchen up for the raw food experience! While you're cleaning, you'll want to identify any equipment that you don't often use or don't need: examples include mini grills, toaster ovens, etc. Find a different place to store these appliances for now or, if you're convinced you won't use them again, donate them or give them away. With what is left, organize your appliances so you have as much space available as possible. After you've gone through this process your kitchen should have a much more minimalist feel. You'll have all the room to prepare your raw foods, with a clean start!

Next, you'll want to pick up some of the raw food staples. If you're just at the start of transitioning to the raw food diet, this will likely mean some simple snacks like nut mixes, dried fruit and vegetable juices. If you're ready to start replacing meals, look up a bunch of different recipes and try to find some ingredients that are common in some or all of them. You can't go wrong with fresh produce, focusing on leafy greens and dark berries. You'll also want to pick up some nuts, seeds, and beans for that irreplaceable protein. If you're almost complete with your transition and have already stocked many of the basics, this is the time to branch out and try some new things. Make sure you sample a lot of super foods such as chia seeds, blueberries, and kale! These foods will form a strong constitution for your diet.

Lastly, you'll want to look into some of the more specialized equipment often found in raw food kitchens.

The absolute most important appliances you'll want to pick up are a water purifier, a juicer, a high speed blender, and a hand blender (the last one is more preference, but it's incredibly convenient). These are appliances that you will find yourself using on a daily basis when you switch to a raw food diet. You'll want to start making your own juice and vegetable shakes as well as purifying your own water as soon as possible. These are easy first steps to get in the swing of what raw food diets are all about. Once you've gotten these necessities, you can start looking into some of the more luxury items for a raw food kitchen. These items include things like coffee grinders (for grinding seeds and nuts), dehydrators, and food processors. While not necessary, many raw-foodies find these appliances indispensable when it comes to preparing more high-quality raw food options.

Equipping your kitchen for your raw food transition can be a big project, but it can also be a ton of fun! Having a space that is conducive to your food choices can make the switch that much easier. When you are switching, cleaning out your kitchen and getting rid of some of your cooking appliances can be a great symbolic way to get into the mental state of your change. Stocking up your kitchen with raw food staples and snacks will be a delightful surprise when you go in the pantry to find out what you're going to eat. Lastly, having access to some nice, high-end appliances will help you solidify your choice in a fun, constructive way!

Chapter 5- Check Out Your Local Food Options

Part of taking on a raw food diet is being conscious about your food's effect on the world and your community. When you buy food from a supermarket, it is almost guaranteed that food has traveled hundreds of miles to get to its destination. This necessitates preservatives in order to keep the food from going bad. These preservatives are not fool-proof, meaning that many foods go bad on the journey; these long-distance food shipments also necessitate waste. Additionally, a large amount of fossil fuels are burned every single day getting food across the country. Eating raw foods is a great way to improve your health and vitality, but it's also a wonderful chance to help improve the health and vitality of the Earth. When you're buying your raw food supplies, check around your local area for farmer's markets and food co-ops. These are excellent choices to buy raw, organic, vegan, and, yes, local alternatives to foods sold at many major supermarkets.

Farmer's markets are a great place to start if you are unsure about where to go to get quality, local raw foods. Many farmer's markets have a wonderful sense of community, and you shouldn't have any trouble finding people who are willing to give you advice on raw foods. Farmer's markets are places where local farmers congregate to sell all manner of goods. Along with the freshest local produce, you'll also be able to find a slew of raw food staples such as raw honey, nuts, seeds, and superfoods. If you're looking for a good place to buy raw food and talk to some like-minded people, look no further than your local farmer's market.

Of course, sometimes, you won't have a farmer's market available to you. In this case, you'll want to look for a local food co-op or a community garden. These resources are usually more accessible, and while they don't offer the all-around community support that a farmer's market might, they are still a great option for picking up raw foods. If your area doesn't have a community garden, start one! Starting a community garden is a rewarding process that can really codify your transition and inspire you to reach for greater and greater heights. If, after some research, you find that starting a community garden is a little too time consuming for your lifestyle, look into starting a personal garden. Much gardening can be done at home, in a yard or on a windowsill. Wheatgrass, for example, is incredibly easy to grow from home. While a personal garden isn't an end-all-be-all resolution for your raw food needs, it can be a wonderful supplement that provides you with some quality produce in exchange for some light labor. For those of you that enjoy gardening already, this is a great option for you!

At the end of the day, your goal should be to make as much of the produce you buy organic and local as possible. Of course, it isn't always reasonable to buy everything from a farmer's market or co-op. Don't worry too much if you have to get some of your goods from the supermarket. Many supermarkets nowadays carry organic and local alternatives. A little bit of research might also suggest that you can find some good places to buy foods outside of where you normally shop. Look around and do your best. Don't let it get you down if you have to get a couple things that aren't organic!

As you'll soon find out, being part of the raw food movement means being conscious about more than just your own health. We greatly encourage you to reach out to your community. Find a farmer's market or co-op and start attending events. Help out at the community garden or start a garden of your own. You'll find that when you surround yourself with a like-minded community, your transition will go much more smoothly. Not only that, but friends are the best way to find the most delicious raw food recipes!

Chapter 6- Moderate and Track Your Nutrition

As we've mentioned in previous chapters, the raw food diet can sometimes be difficult for obtaining certain, specialized vitamins and minerals that come from traditionally cooked and processed foods. When you're transitioning to any new diet, it is important that you slowly introduce your body to the change. By taking things at a reasonable pace, you'll find that you can identify how your body reacts to certain options much better. Everything in moderation rings just as true here as it does for other dietary options! Additionally, until you get the hang of working with your raw food diet, you'll want to monitor your nutritional intake to make sure that you're getting everything you need. Once you get into the swing of things, you'll be experiencing nutrition, health, and vitality like you've never felt before, but at the start it's important to make sure you set the right standards for

31

yourself. Many people tend to overdo the fruits and leafy greens for example, shunning nuts and beans, and therefore developing vitamin deficiencies. Even though you're eating only raw food, variety is still king.

Moderation and careful tracking of your food intake will help make your transition smooth, painless, and fun!

When transitioning to a raw food diet, there are a couple of golden rules that you can't go wrong with following. The first is to drink plenty of water! This hasn't changed from any other diet you might have practiced. Water is incredibly important for your bodies, but also for detoxification and weight loss. This is why a water purifier is an essential for your kitchen. Many places, especially big cities, have heavily treated tap water that doesn't mix well with the raw food diet's principles. Filter your water and drink a good amount a day! Aim for six to eight normally sized glasses. By regulating your water intake, you'll make sure you'll have a solid foundation for building the rest of your raw food habits.

When you're starting off, make sure to eat a ton of dark, leafy greens. These are the types of vegetables that tend to have the most vitamin and mineral densities, with some vegetables like kale even being hailed as superfoods. These foods should help form the core of your diet and will slingshot your health and vitality to unprecedented heights. Additionally, make sure you don't overdo it with fruits. While fruits are a wonderful snack or addition to a well-rounded meal, they are very sugary and don't provide the hearty substance that other foods will. Keep fruits around, of course, but don't think that a raw food diet means you can just eat fruit and be good! Lastly, you're going to want to rely on beans, nuts, and lentils to get a good amount of protein. Protein is sometimes difficult to obtain for vegetarians and vegans, and these handy foods are the solution. Always keep some around and make sure you have a source of protein with each meal and even with snacks.

Even with all of these steps, you may still want to consider taking a dietary supplement. Children especially should be given supplementary treatments for the potential lack of vitamin b12 and vitamin D that come with the diet. A daily multivitamin should be enough for most adults, but be sure to consult with a dietician before fully transitioning to a raw food diet to see how you can take the most advantage of your new nutritional options.

The main idea here is variety and careful selection. As long as you make sure you're not stagnating on one or two foods, you should benefit from increased nutrition, health, and vitality. You can bolster this even more by taking a supplement. Water and a wide variety of options will spell good health before you know it! As long as you indulge in moderation and do your best to track what you're eating, you'll soon fall back into habit. Once eating raw becomes second nature, the true benefits of this amazing diet will start to show.

Chapter 7- Keep Up the Exercise!

Now, I know what you're thinking: "this has nothing to do with raw food!" But that simply isn't true! The choice of transitioning to a raw food diet is one with health at the epicenter. Everything that surrounds the decision to transfer to raw food leads back to one's health. You can do everything perfectly as this book describes and eat things that are only strictly raw and vegan, but if you don't supplement those choices with an active lifestyle, you will not achieve the health that you desire. This is especially true if you're looking to transition to raw food in order to lose weight or detoxify your body. Raw foods, simply put, are most helpful with an active lifestyle. Not only that, but a lot of the foods you'll consume in a raw diet, such as nut mixes and vegetable shakes, are the perfect complement to a good workout!

When you're transitioning to a raw food lifestyle, there will be three main categories that many people will find they need work on: the food itself, the community aspect, and exercise. All three of these factors are necessary to gain the most from a raw food diet. We've discussed the food and the community in past chapters. This chapter, we'll focus on some exercise ideas.

If you're already set in an exercise routine, then you'll probably be fine staying with that routine during your transition. The only thing you'll want to keep in mind is that if your workouts are intense, like cross-country running or bodybuilding, this diet might not be right for you. Those exercise options are amazing for the right kind of people, but they often necessitate a very special and usually incredibly high-protein variety of diets. This section is aimed more toward people who lead a sedentary lifestyle or don't exercise as much as they would like.

To start, you should start a walking regimen. Walking is a wonderful pastime that isn't too straining and can even be fun! Start by walking for 30 minutes a day. Feel free to take one day off a week if you must, but it is best to walk a bit every day. This is on top of any walking that you might be doing anyway. Use this walking to clear your mind, almost like mediation. Set yourself up on a schedule and stick with it!

Once you've gotten in the hang of dedicating a small amount of time to walking each day, then you'll want to step up your game. A great way to get exercise that will also likely help you meet people in the vegan, organic and raw food communities is yoga. Look around your town or city and see if there is any yoga classes offered. Yoga is a relaxed, extended series of stretching exercises that is very relaxing and great for your health. It increases longevity, reduces stress, and is beneficial to your overall health- the perfect complement to a raw food diet! If you can't find a class near you, there are plenty of wonderful guides online you can find. Consider starting up a class or meet-up yourself! Again, part of the transition is finding a good community to help you out. Once you've gotten used to yoga, some people like to move on to some more intense regiments like Pilates. How intense you would like to go is up to you, but you'd like to aim for something like 10 hours of exercise a week. This will get you into shape and jumpstart the active lifestyle that is paired best with your raw food diet.

Conclusion

Thank you again for downloading this book!

I hope this book was able to help you to transition smoothly into a raw food diet

The next step is to keep up the good work and keep in touch with your local communities! Give back where you can and teach some other interested people the benefits of a raw food diet.

Finally, if you enjoyed this book, then I'd like to ask you for a favor, would you be kind enough to leave a review for this book on Amazon? It'd be greatly appreciated!

Click here to leave a review for this book on Amazon!

Thank you and good luck!